blessed yogi

A Coloring Book by Shades for the Soul

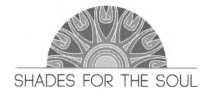

SHADES FOR THE SOUL

ISBN-978-0-9944266-0-4

Shades for the Soul books is in Brisbane, Australia.

The book is written by Corene Gavin and Anna Trivedi in collaboration with artists and designers.
The copyright © belongs to Shades for the Soul as of 2015. We reserve all rights.

Shades for the Soul

We created this book to soothe your mind so that your beautiful soul
can shine more brightly. Drawing on Vedic and Buddhist teachings
and the graceful beauty of yoga, we have gathered illustrations and
patterns to calm your busy mind and enliven your spirit.

We would love to see how you bring these illustrations to life with
your own shades! Share your work with the Shades for the Soul
community, and follow us for inspiration, recommendations
and suggestions on how to use color.

shadesforthesoul.com

Instagram.com/shadesforthesoul

Facebook.com/shadesforthesoul

Pinterest.com/shadesforthesoul

@shadesbooks

How to get the most out of this book

A calm mind is a fertile, creative mind. Coloring is deeply restful and soothing, and is a great way to re-set your mind to its natural calm state.

To enhance your experience using this book we recommend:

1. Turning off your phone and take a few cleansing, deep breaths.

2. Smile.

3. Put on some music that suits your mood.

4. Flick through the book until an image grabs your attention.

5. Begin coloring.

6. Allow yourself to settle into the process of intuitively selecting colors, and let your mind wander freely and easily.

7. You may find that new ideas and solutions to problems come to you as you color. Jot your thoughts or inspirational ideas down on the blank pages next to the illustration.

8. Continue as long as you feel the flow of creative energy moving through you. Any time is a good time to finish.

May we exist like the lotus,
at ease in muddy water.

Unknown

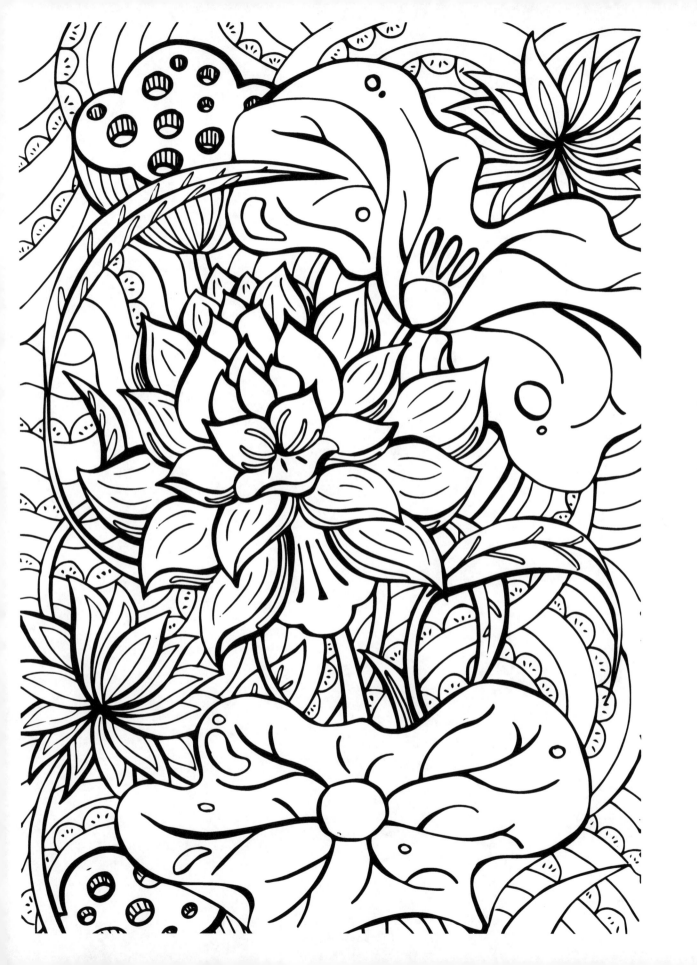

Close your eyes.
Clear your heart.
Let it go.

Unknown

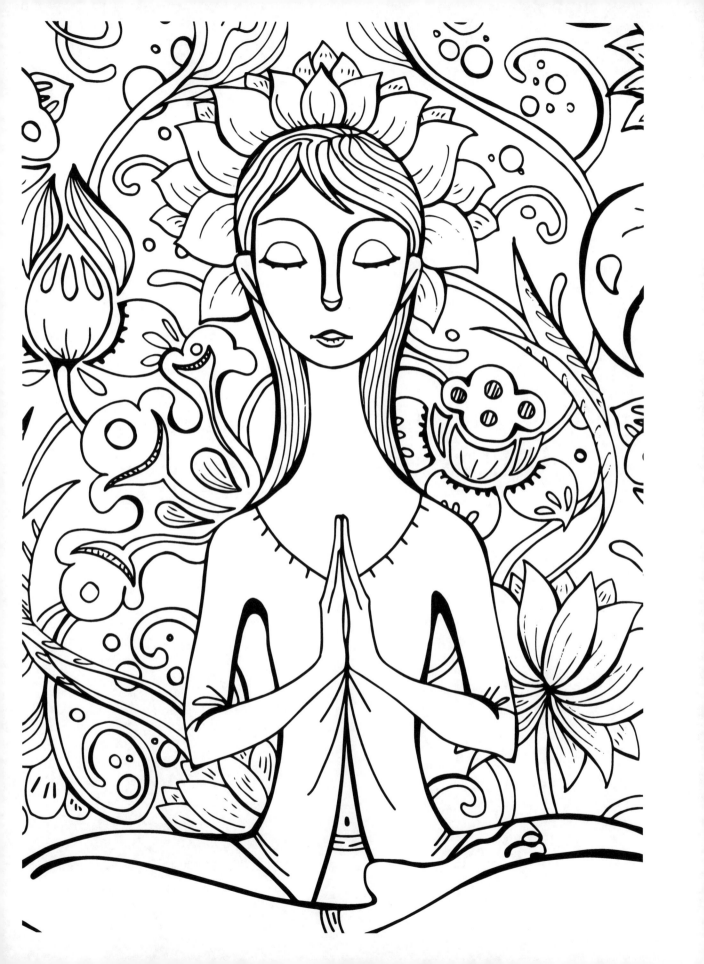

We can never obtain peace in the outer world until we make peace with ourselves.

Dalai Lama

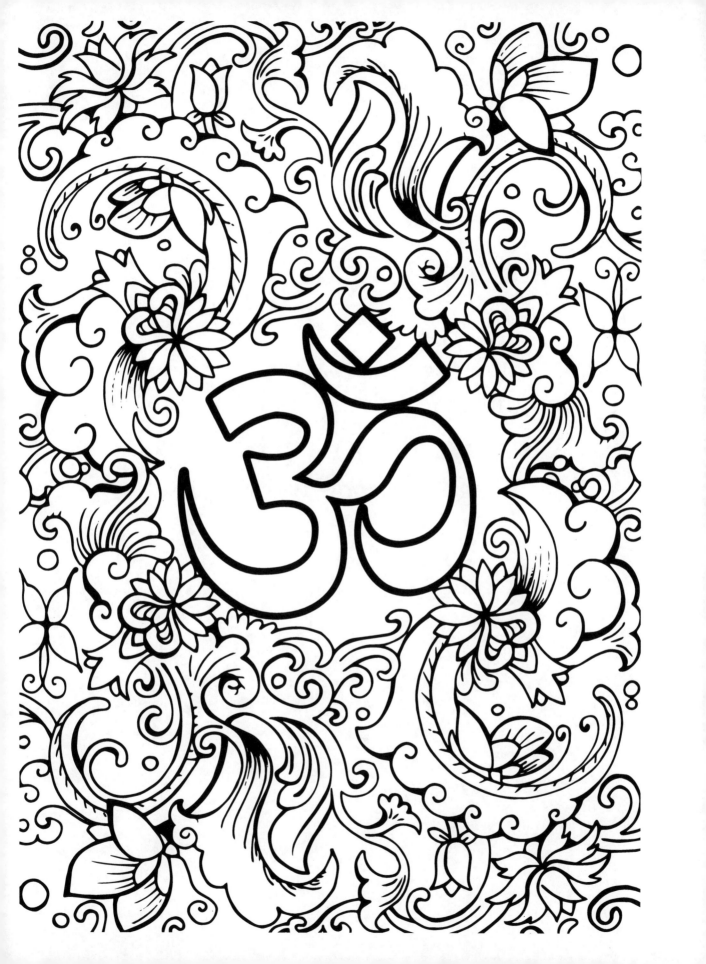

I found things I could say with color and shapes
that I couldn't say any other way —
things I had now had words for.

Georgia O'Keefe

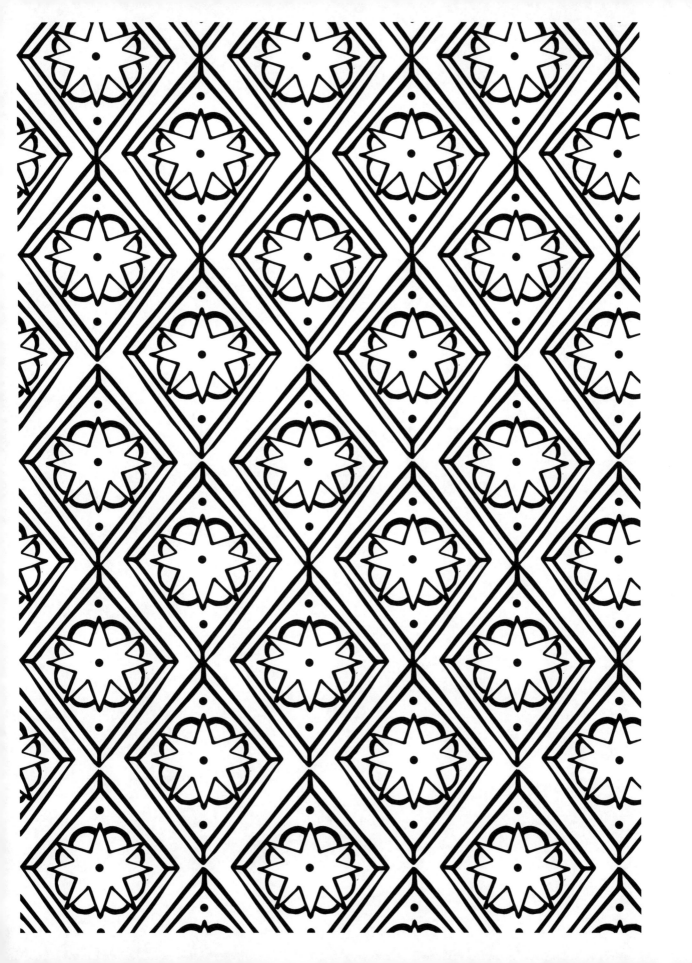

What we achieve inwardly
will change outer reality.

Plutarch

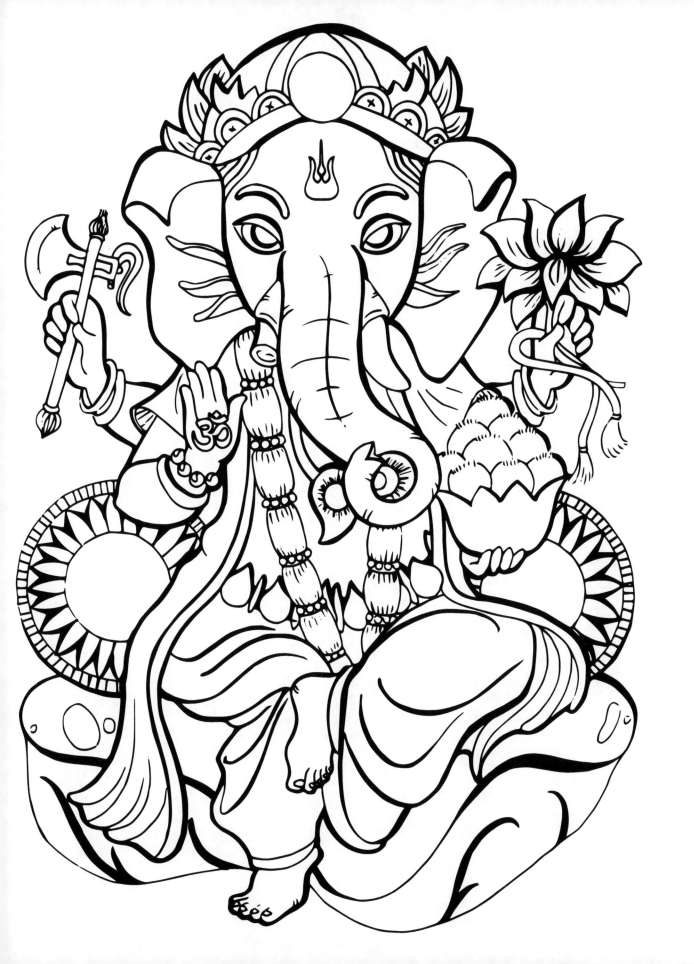

Colors are the smiles of nature.

James Henry Leigh Hunt

The longest journey of any person
is the journey inward.

Unknown

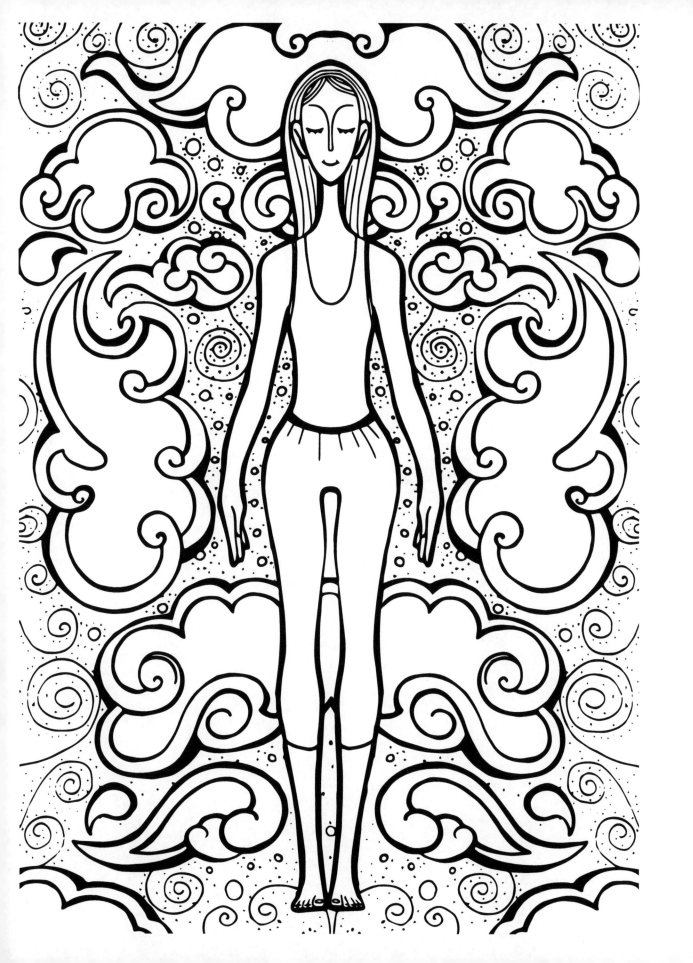

Life is like an ever-shifting kaleidoscope —
a slight change, and all patterns alter.

Sharon Salzberg

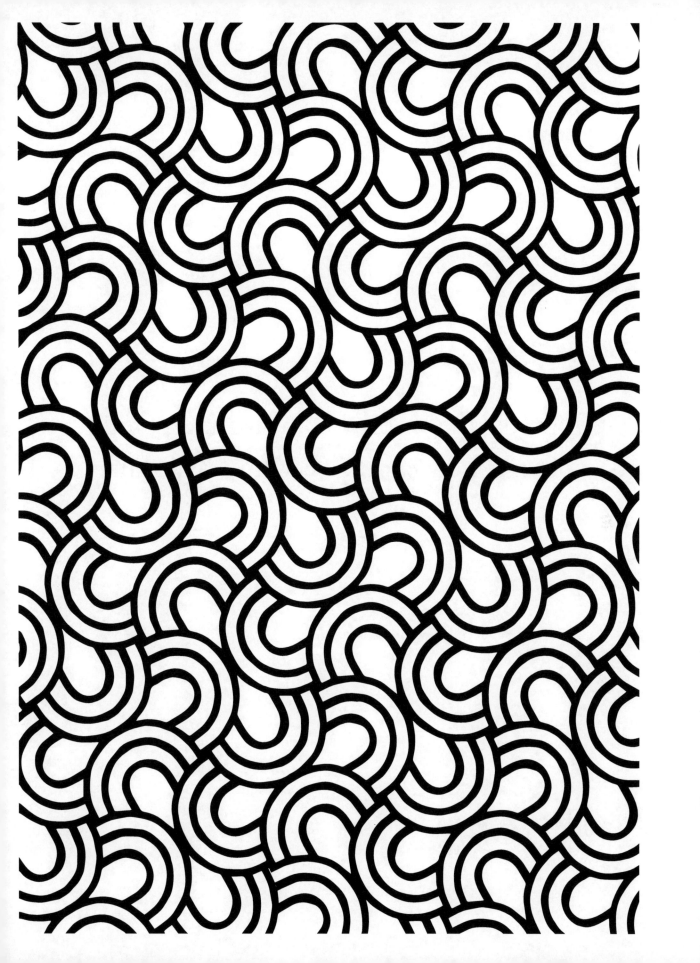

Amidst the worldly comings and goings,
observe how endings become beginnings.

Tao Te Ching

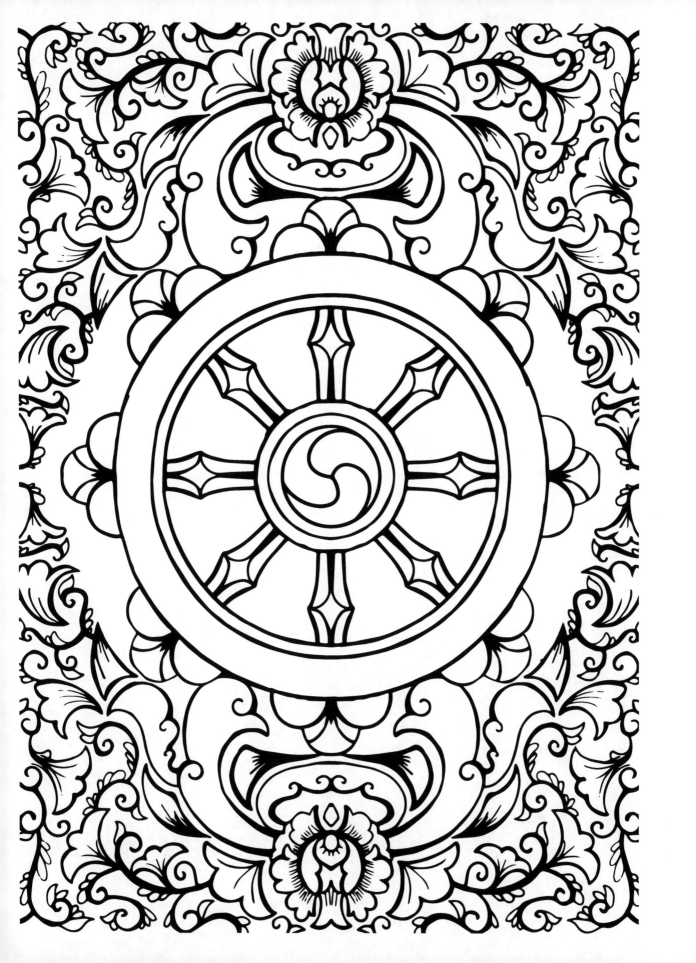

The sun shines not on us but in us.

John Muir

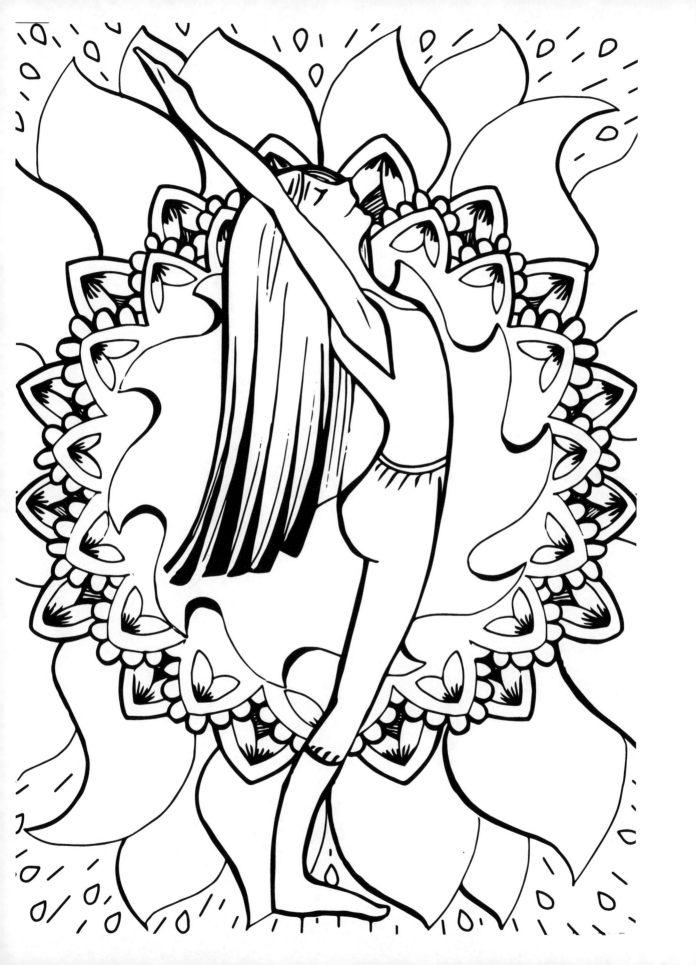

The quieter you become,
the more you can hear.

Ram Dass

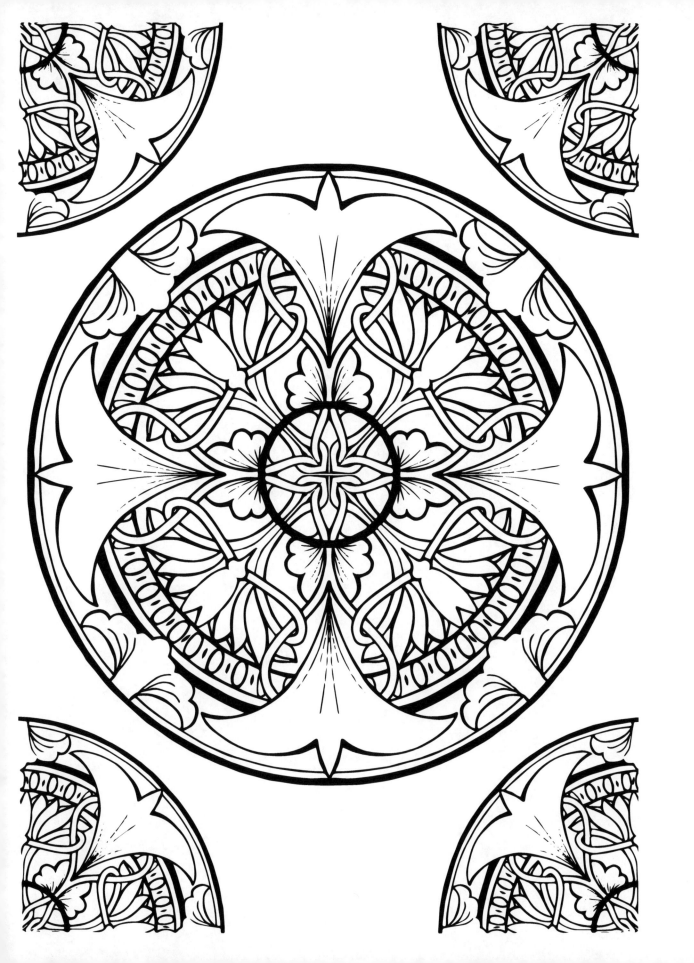

Color is the fruit of life.

Guillaume Apollinaire

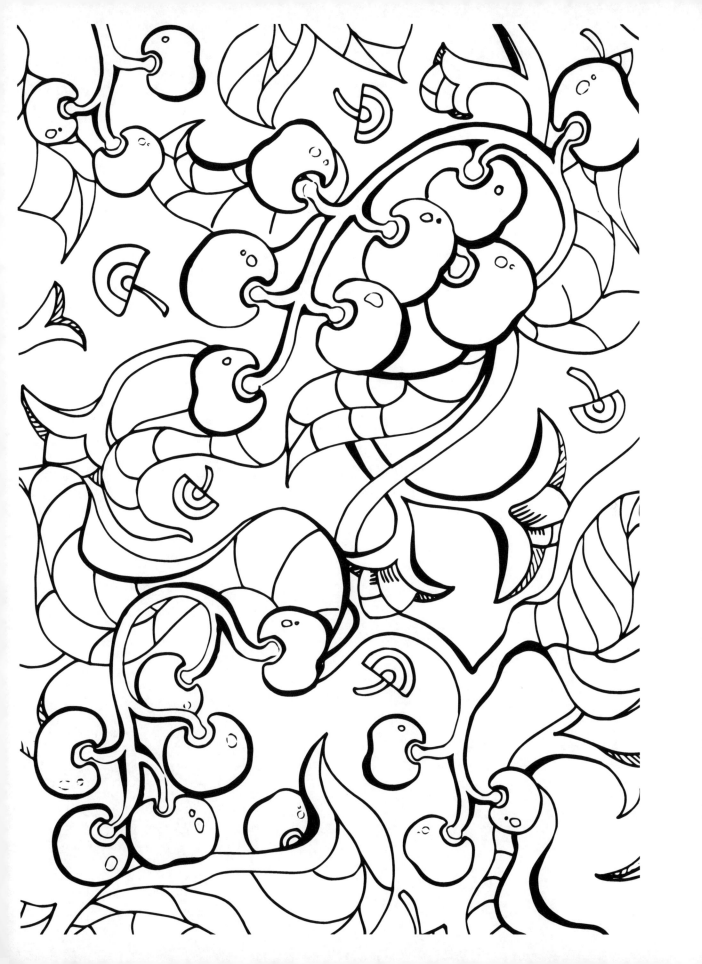

Life shrinks or expands
in proportion to one's courage.

Anaïs Nin

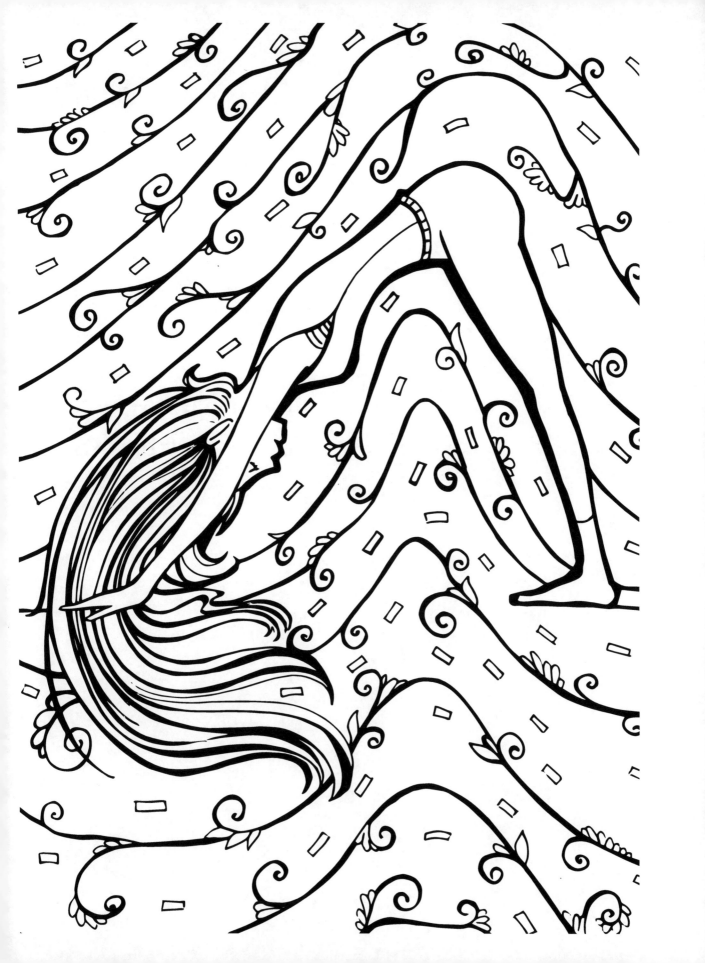

All we have is all we need.
All we need is the awareness of how blessed
we really are.

Sarah Ban Breathnach

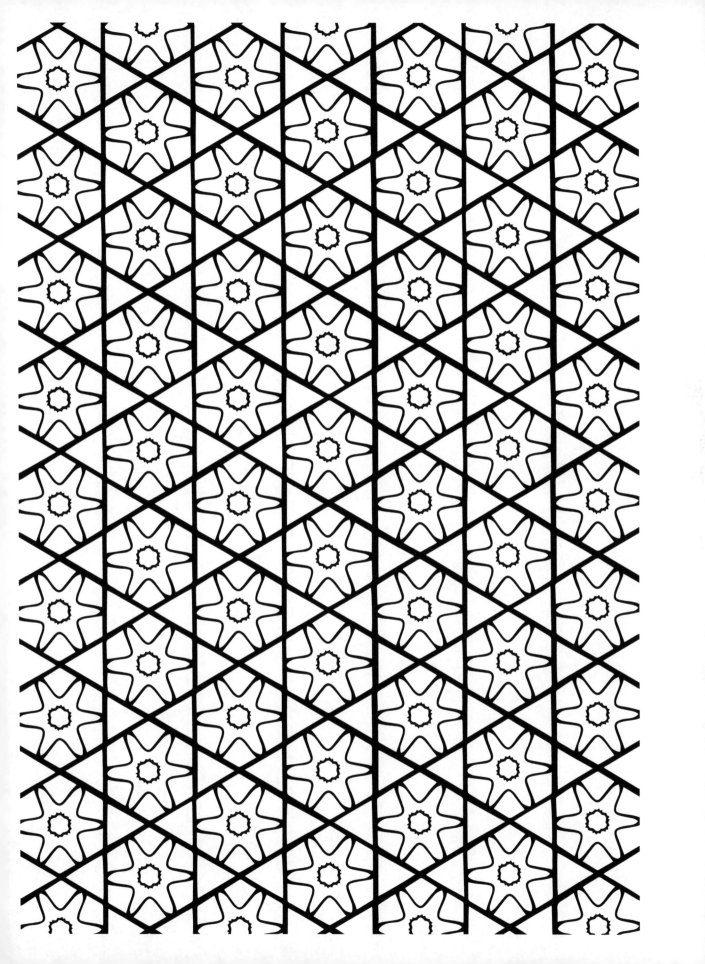

Do not feel lonely,
the entire universe is within you.

Rumi

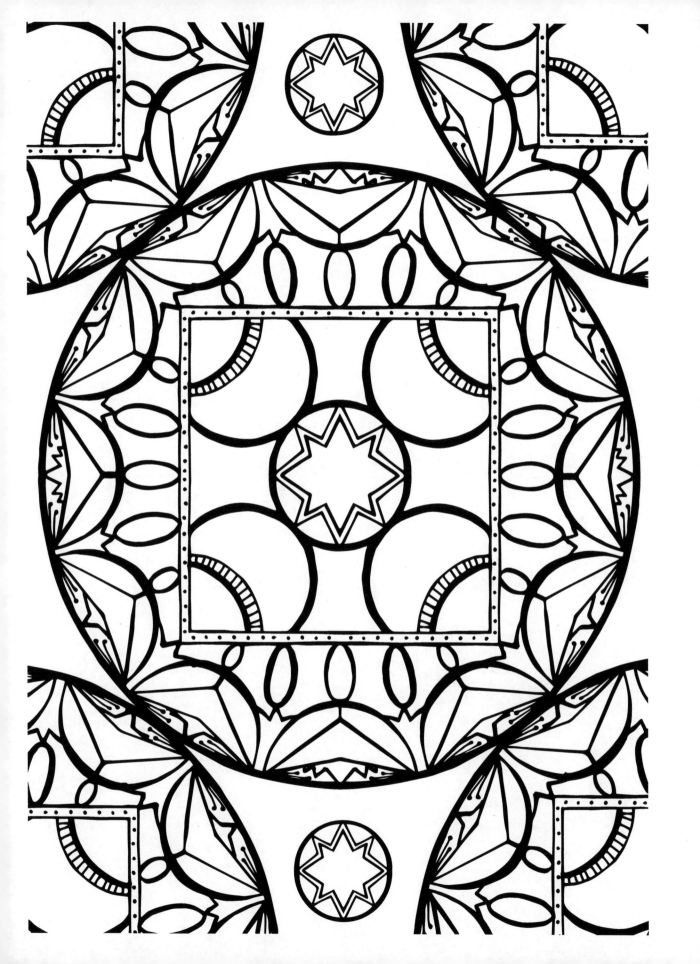

You are the sky.
Everything else – it's just weather.

Pema Chödrön

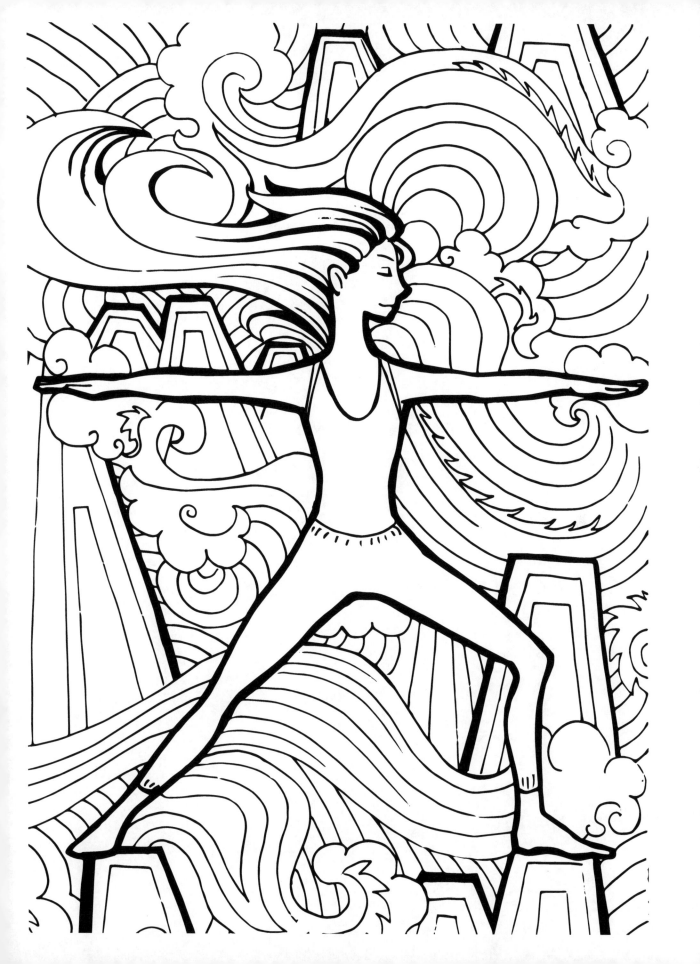

Color is power which directly
influences the soul.

Wassily Kandinsky

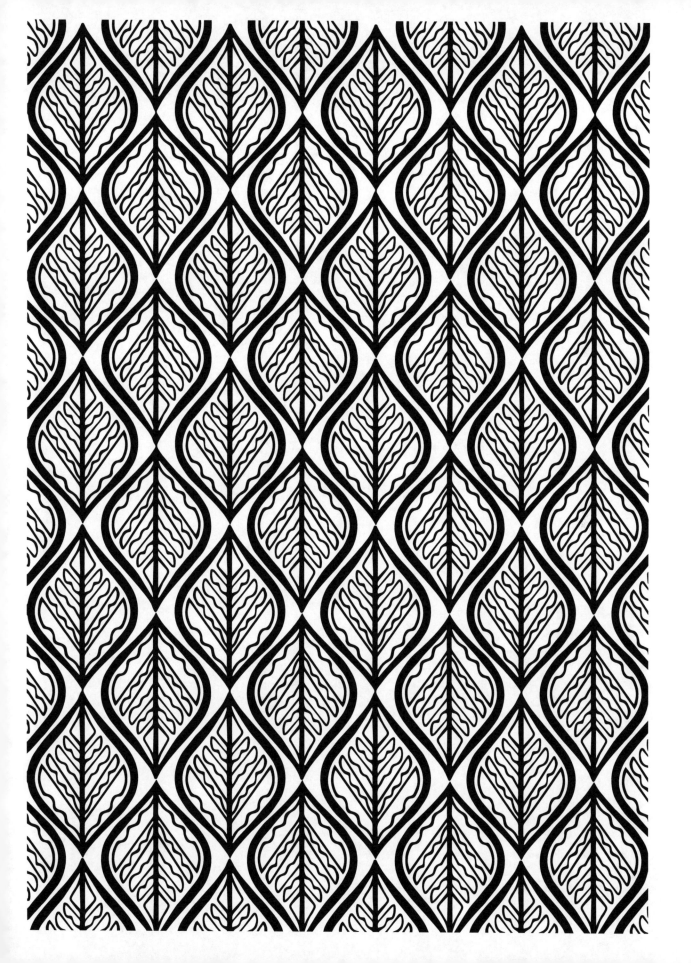

Happiness is when what you think,
what you say, and what you do
are in harmony.

Mahatma Ghandi

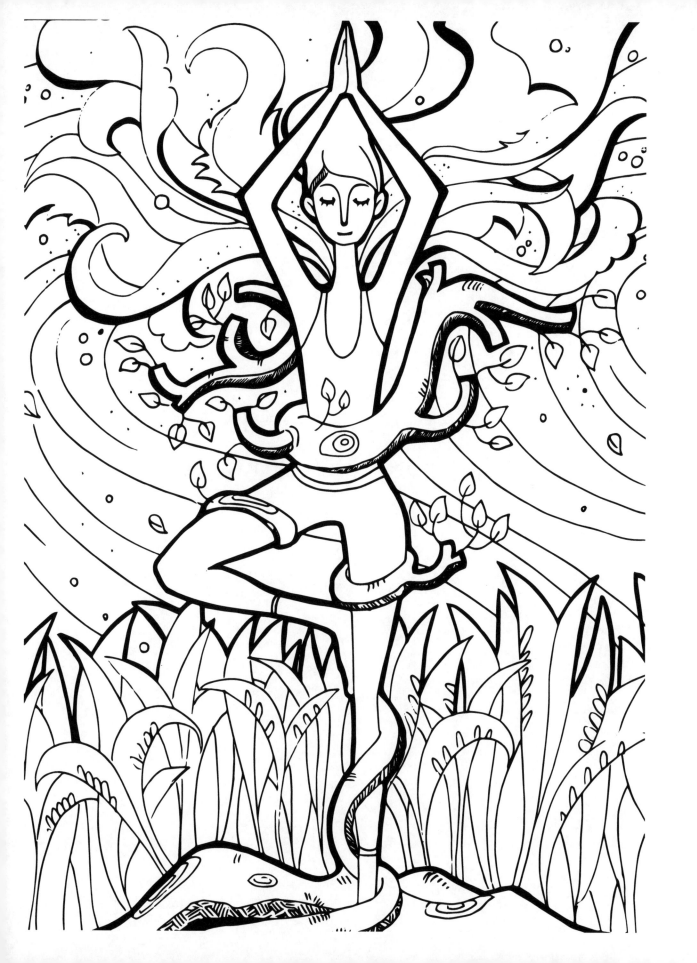

I see my life as an unfolding set of opportunities to awaken.

Ram Dass

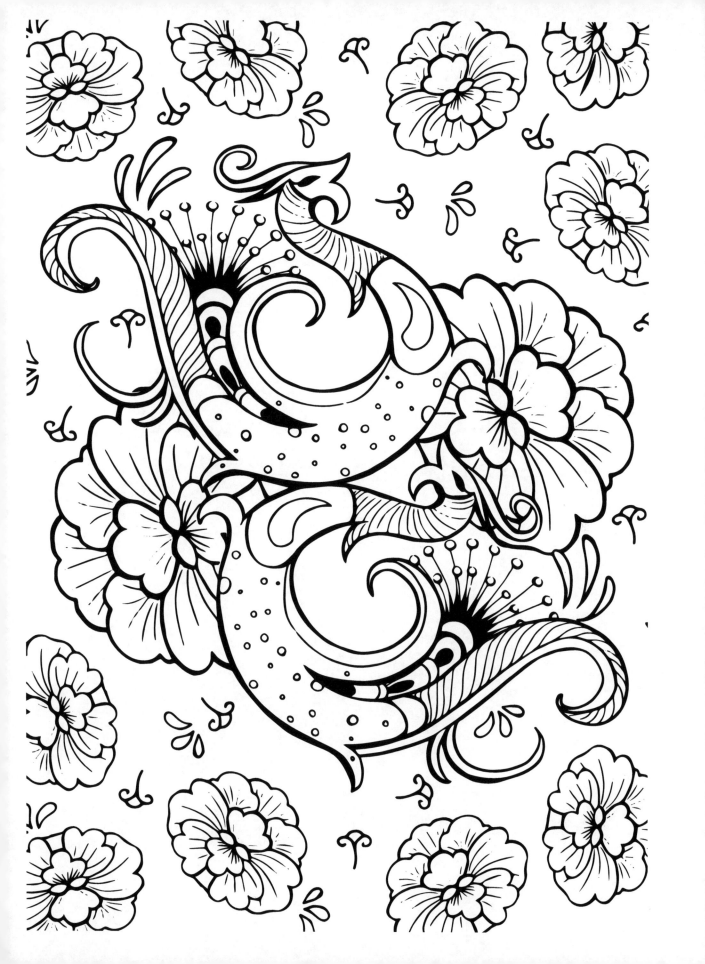

It is not joy that makes us grateful;
it is gratitude that makes us joyful.

Brother David Steidl Rost

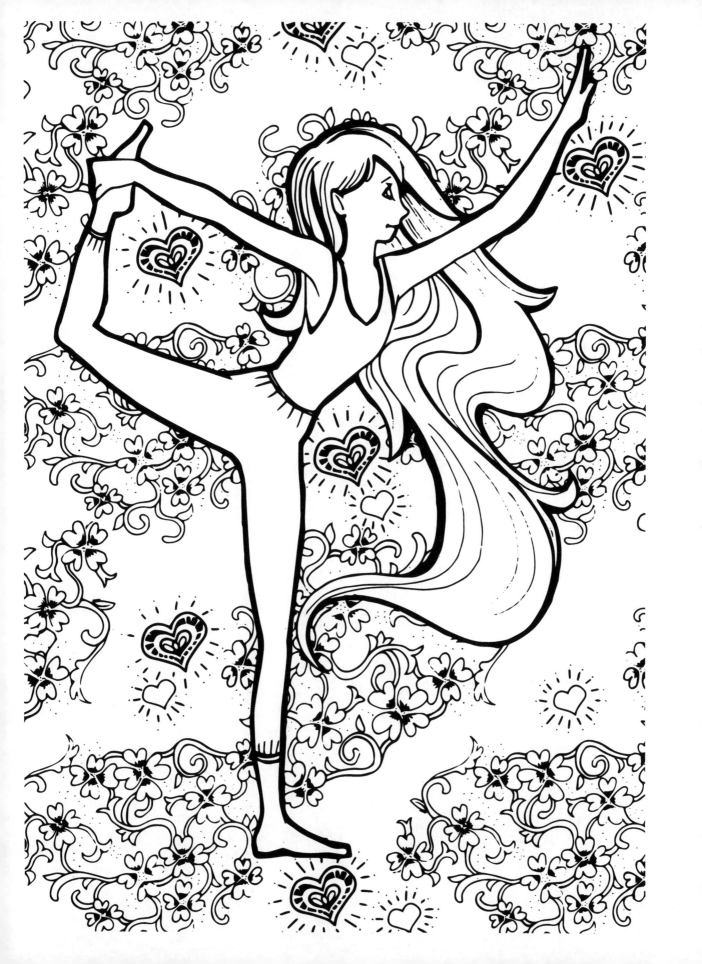

Color is like the mother tongue
of the subconscious.

Carl Jung

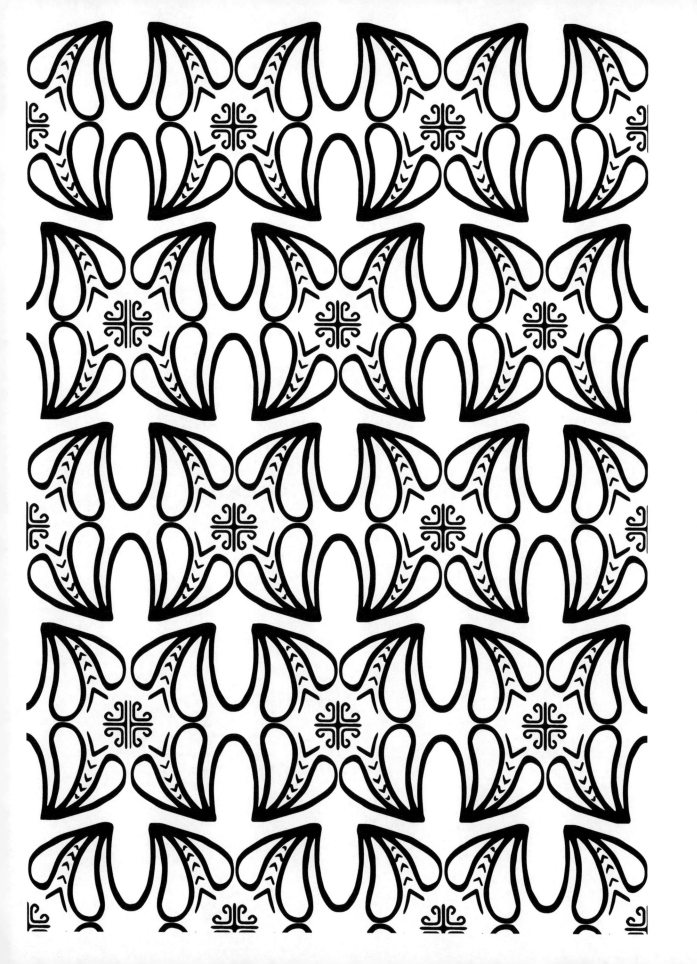

Only when we are brave enough
to explore the darkness will we discover
the infinite power of our light.

Brené Brown

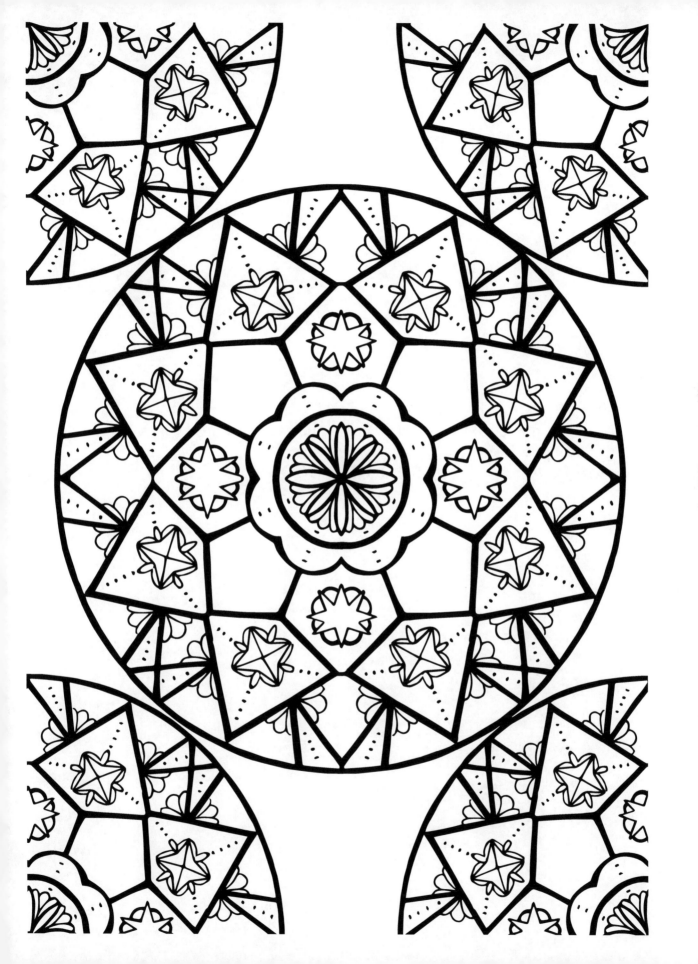

The creation of a thousand forests
is in one acorn.

Ralph Waldo Emerson

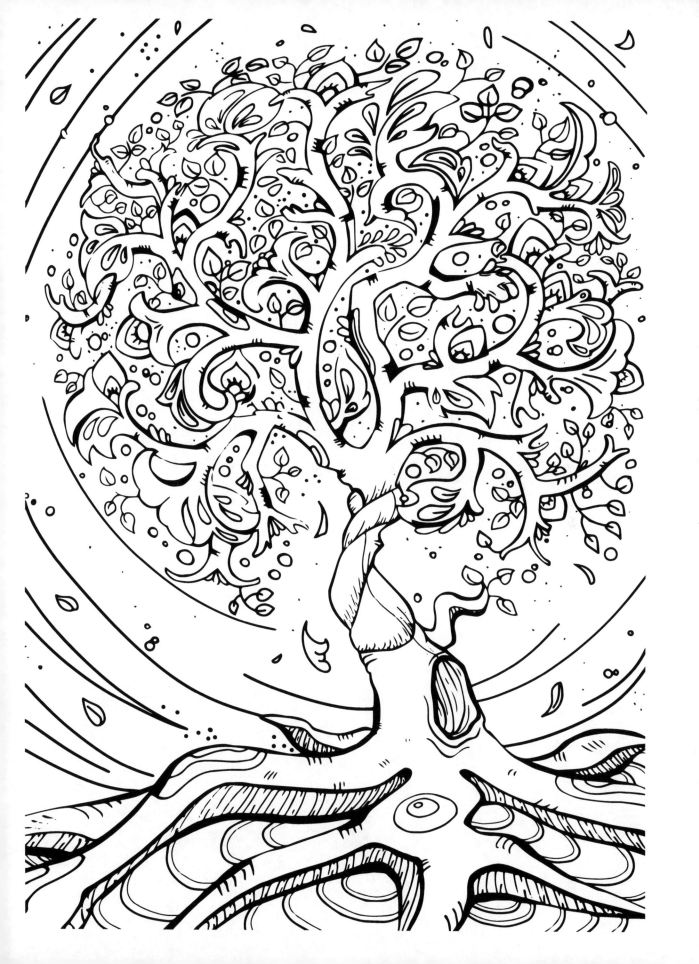

Nature does not hurry,
yet everything gets accomplished.

Lao Tzu

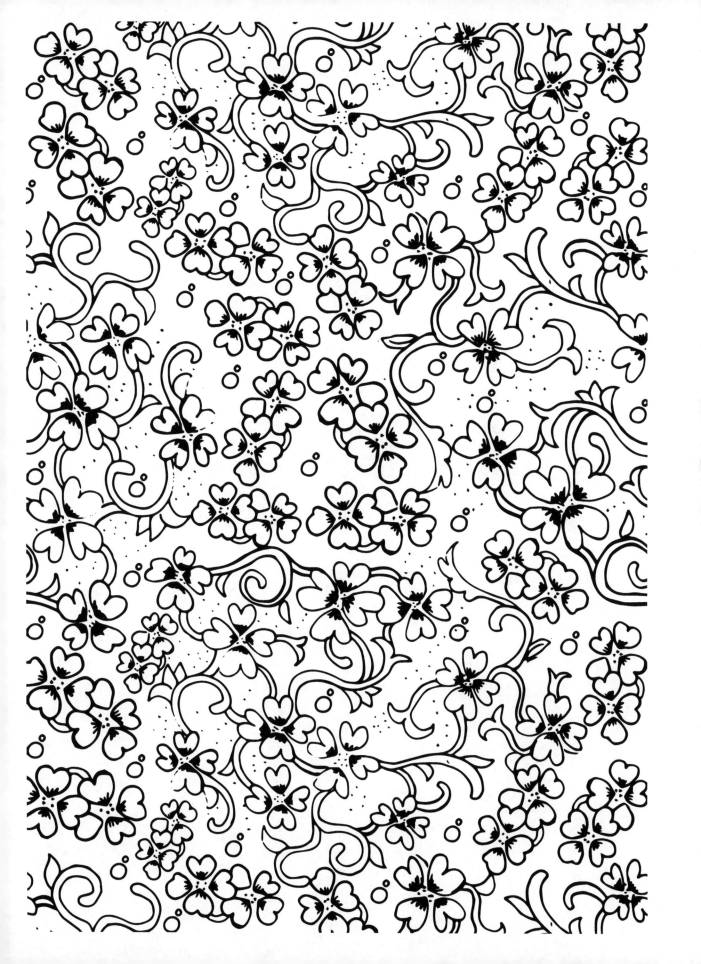

Be gentle with yourself.
You are a child of the universe,
no less than the trees and the stars;
you have a right to be here.

Max Ehrmann

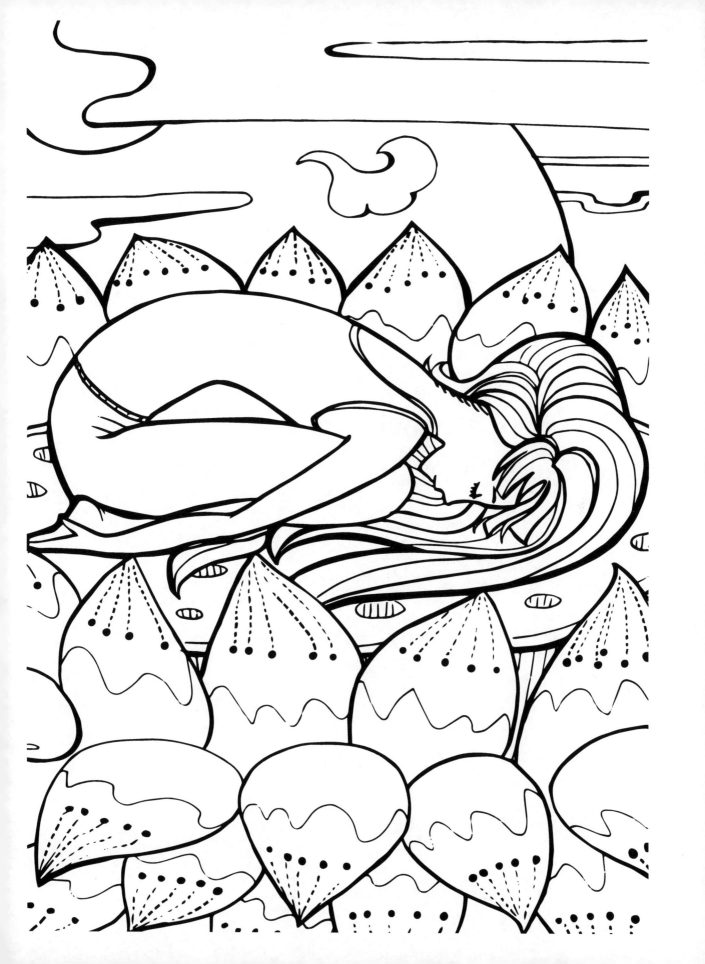

The soul becomes dyed
with the color of its thoughts.

Marcus Aurelius

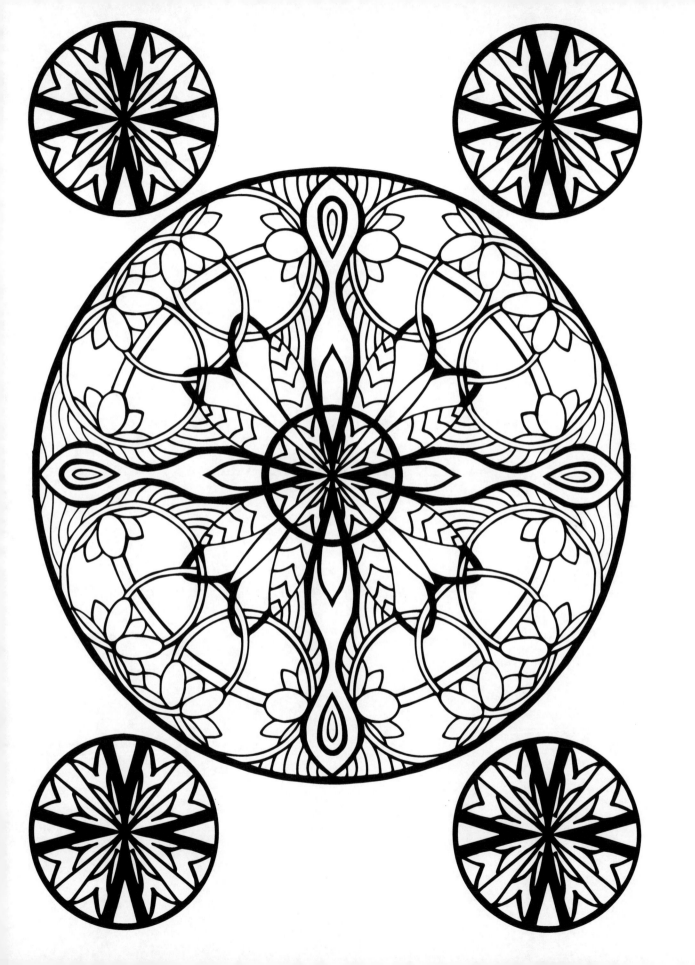

There is no way to happiness —
happiness is the way.

Thich Nhat Hanh

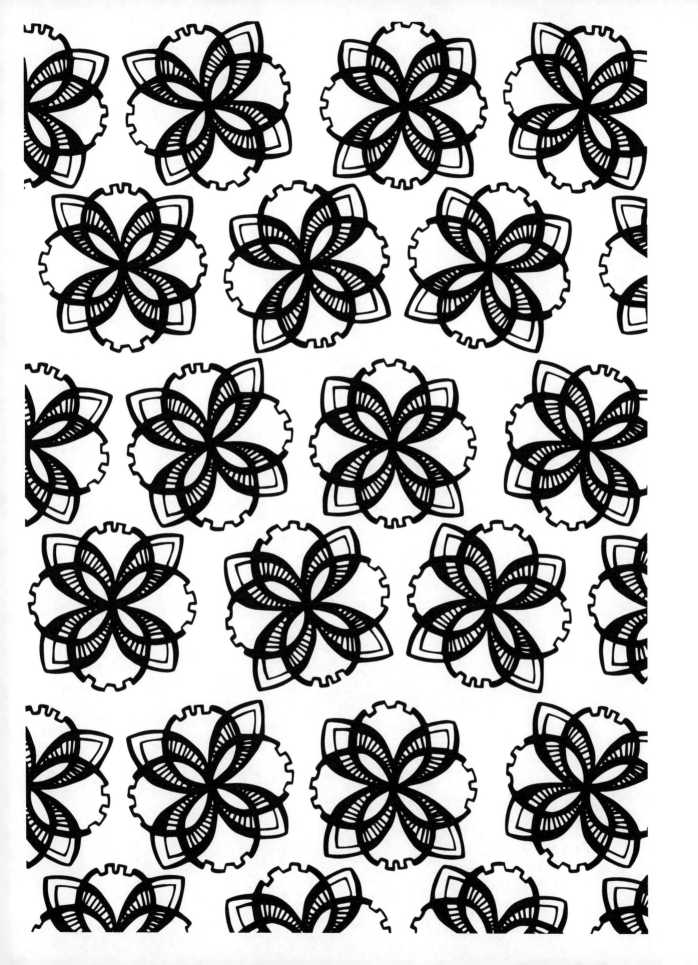

Hope is the thing with feathers
That perches in the soul
And sings the tune without the words
And never stops at all

Emily Dickinson

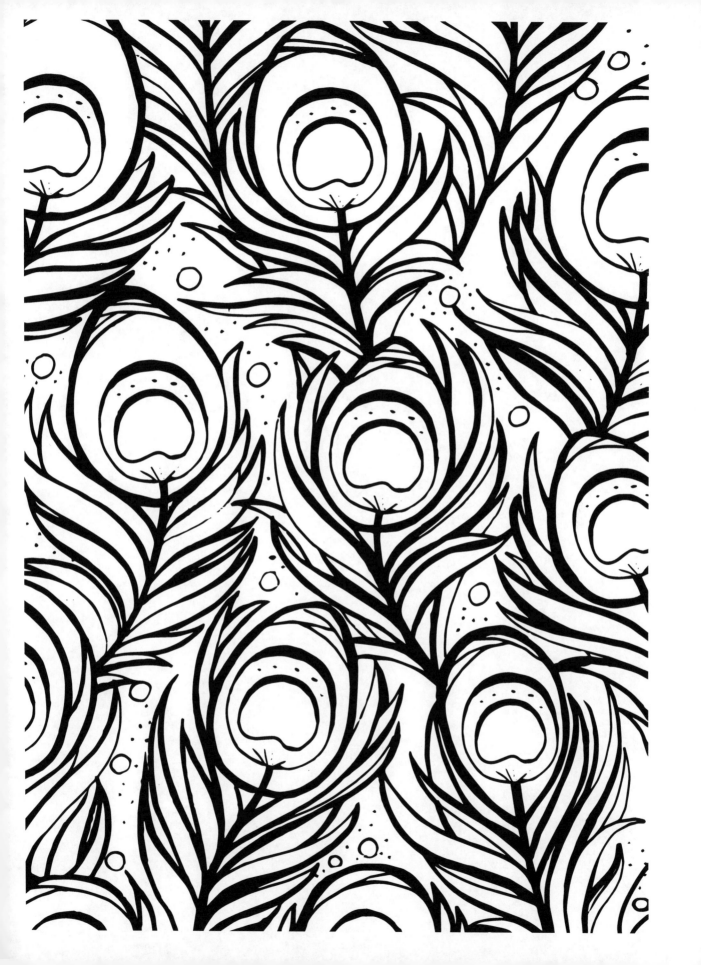

Life is a balance
of holding on
and letting go.

Unknown

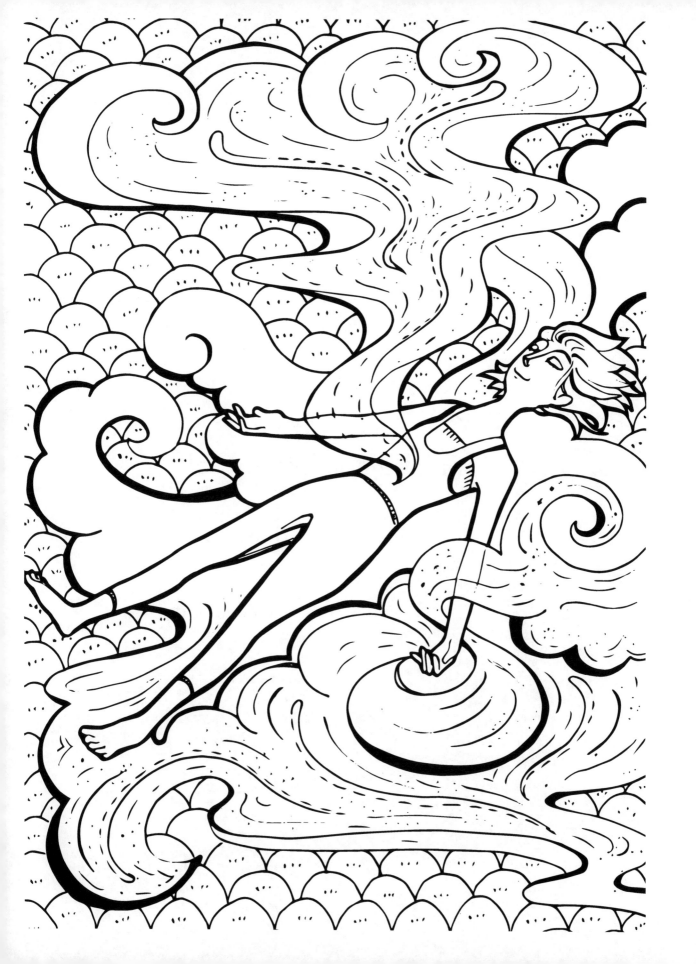

Yoga is the journey of the self,
through the self, to the self.

The Bhagavad Gita

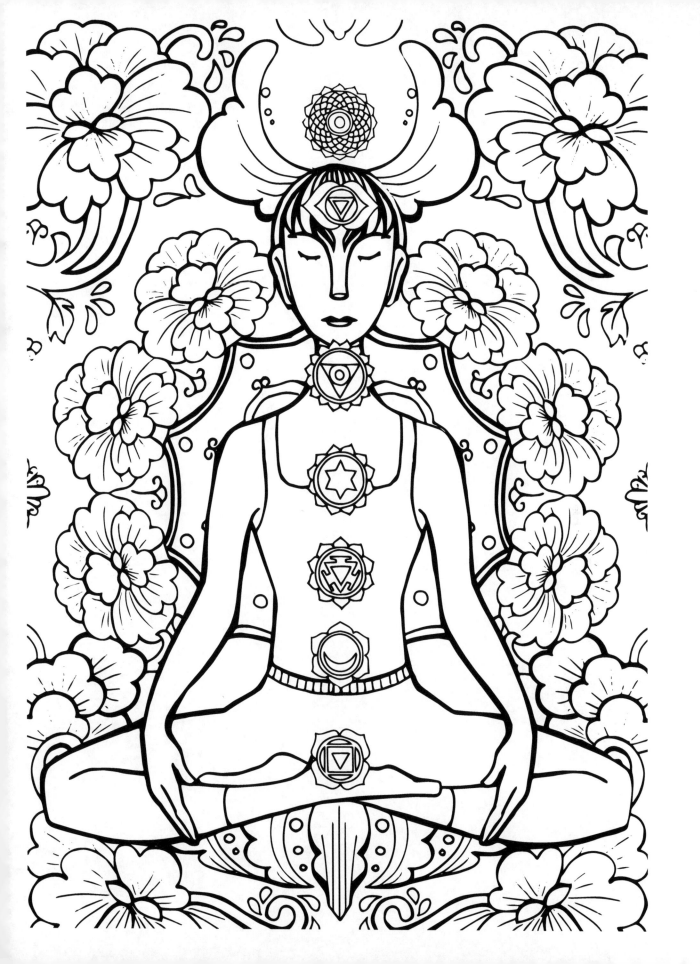

Made in the USA
Middletown, DE
12 November 2015